The Pocket Guide to Hysterectomy

by
Linda Parkinson-Hardman

First edition published by:
The Hysterectomy Association
www.hysterectomy-association.org.uk

ISBN 978-0-9532445-9-1

Contents

PREFACE

Within this guide you will find information on the operation, the menopause, hormone replacement therapy (HRT), natural alternatives to hormone replacement therapy, support groups and information sources as well as some information about related physical issues such as osteoporosis.

Hysterectomy is, by its very nature, a turning point in many women's lives and for the vast majority it will be a positive event, ending possibly years of distressing gynaecological symptoms. This booklet does, of necessity, include information about most of the possible outcomes, both positive and negative, associated with hysterectomy. However, most women will experience few, if any, of the problems highlighted and in those cases where there are difficulties, it is highly improbable that anyone would experience all of them.

DISCLAIMER

Although much of this book represents current medical opinion, some of the information and resources listed in this book are by definition, outside the scope of generally accepted medical standards of care. They may be non-conventional, alternative or complementary.

The information and resources listed should not be used in any way to provide a diagnosis or to prescribe any medical treatment. As in the case of conventional medicine, indiscriminate use of some therapies presented, without medical supervision may be harmful to your health. Individuals reading this material should in all cases, consult their own doctor or health practitioner for the diagnosis and treatment of medical conditions. The author and publisher cannot accept responsibility for illness arising out of failure to seek medical advice from a doctor.

INTRODUCTION

Almost 60,000 hysterectomy operations were carried out on women in the UK in 2011/2012. It can, and does, help to ease many gynaecological complaints, including heavy and/or painful periods and endometriosis. It is rarely performed for reasons of saving life, but it can be a permanent cure for some gynaecological cancers.

The majority of hysterectomies are performed when a woman is aged between 40–50 but many do occur before and after this age group. Women, who have a hysterectomy that removes their ovaries, as well as other organs, will go through the menopause immediately after the operation regardless of their age (if they haven't already). Women who have a hysterectomy that leaves one or both of their ovaries intact have a 50% chance of going through the menopause within two to five years of their operation, again regardless of their age, if they haven't already.

WHAT IS A HYSTERECTOMY?

Hysterectomy is the surgical removal of the uterus (uterus). It is one of the most common of all surgical procedures for women in the UK. It can also involve the removal of part of the vagina, the fallopian tubes, ovaries and cervix to cure or help a number of gynaecological complaints. Following this operation you will no longer have periods, you will not be fertile and you will not be able to have any more children.

There are two main ways to perform a hysterectomy. The most common way is to remove the uterus through a cut in the lower abdomen, the second, less common, way is to remove only the uterus through a cut in the top of the vagina, the top of vagina is then stitched. Each operation lasts for up to two hours and is performed, in hospital, usually under a general anaesthetic.

The type of hysterectomy that you have will depend upon the condition it is being used to treat.

- A "total hysterectomy" removes the uterus and cervix. It requires a four to eight inch cut in the abdomen, which may be vertical if there is a large mass (fibroids for instance) to remove.
- A "subtotal hysterectomy" (Laparoscopic Supra-cervical Hysterectomy) removes the uterus but leaves the cervix in place. It is possible that it may help in maintaining a

woman's sexual response as well as help to prevent any future prolapse; however research in this area is inconclusive at the moment. If you have this operation you will need to continue to have smear tests.

- A "total hysterectomy with bilateral (both) or unilateral (one) salpingo-oopherectomy" removes the uterus, cervix, fallopian tubes and both or one of the ovaries.

- A Wertheim's hysterectomy removes the uterus, cervix, part of the vagina, fallopian tubes, peritoneum (this is the broad band of ligament below the uterus), the lymph glands and fatty tissue of the pelvis and possibly one or both ovaries. A Wertheim's hysterectomy is usually performed where cancer is suspected or known to be present.

- Vaginal Hysterectomy. The surgeon operates entirely through the vagina, pulling the uterus down through the vagina into view, disconnecting the cervix and then the rest of the uterus. It is not suitable for all conditions requiring a hysterectomy, such as those requiring removal of the ovaries and/or large fibroids. Generally the woman must also have a fairly loose vagina (usually from having had children) as this widens and relaxes the vagina and connections to the uterus, making them easier to pull through. There is no abdominal scar and it may require a shorter stay in hospital and a quicker recovery period. Vaginal hysterectomy is a preferred route if all the specific requirements are met. The risk factors associated with this type of surgery occasionally relate to an increased risk of developing stress incontinence in later life.

- Laparoscopically Assisted Vaginal hysterectomy (LAH). This is a relatively new procedure that uses keyhole surgery to insert a small viewing instrument into the abdomen. The surgeon can then remove the uterus or ovaries if required through the vagina. The small incisions leave the woman with minimal scarring which should reduce recovery time to 6-8 weeks. However, the operation takes longer to perform and there is a greater risk of complications, which may result in this procedure not being made widely available in the future. LAVH is performed on women who can have a vaginal hysterectomy but who also need the ovaries removed; or who have had surgery previously which might make the vaginal route alone more risky and therefore less successful, for instance in those who have cancer or large fibroids. The vagina must still be loose and open.

WHY MIGHT YOU NEED THIS OPERATION?

Hysterectomy may sometimes become necessary for the following medical reasons:

- Cancer of the uterus, ovaries, fallopian tube/s or cervix
- Endometriosis caused by tissues that normally form inside the uterus forming outside the uterus in the abdominal cavity.
- Fibroids which cause pain, bleeding or are very large. A fibroid is a non-cancerous growth of muscle and fibrous tissue.
- Heavy vaginal bleeding or bleeding that is irregular or very painful
- Pelvic inflammatory disease or adhesions which have pain that is not controlled by other means.
- Prolapse of the uterus, where the uterus falls into the vagina.
- Emergencies, if there is significant gynaecological bleeding which cannot be stopped by any other means.

A hysterectomy may be recommended if none of the other treatments for these conditions has been successful. Some of the conditions may clear up of their own accord, for instance following the menopause or after you have had a D&C operation (Dilation and Curettage where the lining of the uterus is scraped away and if necessary examined).

Cancer of the Reproductive System   There are six main cancer's of the female reproductive organs; cancer of the uterus, cancer of the fallopian tubes, cervical cancer, ovarian cancer, cancer of the vagina and cancer of the vulva.

Cancer of the uterus (endometrial cancer) starts in the lining of the endometrium and may then spread to the fallopian tubes, ovaries and the lymphatic system. The symptoms may include bleeding between periods or spotting if you have already gone through the menopause. There may also be a pink to brown discharge and intermittent period-like pains. It is the fifth most common cancer amongst women and it occurs mainly in women between the aged of 50 and 60 who have not had children. Unfortunately there are no early detection tests for this type of cancer, however as the cancer grows very slowly, it is essential that any symptoms are reported as early as possible.

Cancer of the fallopian tubes is very rare, it accounts for around 0.1 to 0.5% of all gynaecological cancers. Patients may have a watery vaginal discharge, pelvic pain, vaginal bleeding and a small lump. The cancer grows very slowly and as bleeding occurs quite early on it is usually easy to detect and remove before it spreads to the lymph nodes and ovaries.

Cervical cancer can develop in women who have changes in the cells of the cervix; this is why it is important to ensure that regular smear tests are carried out. The main symptoms are a watery, bloody discharge which may smell and bleeding between periods or after the menopause or after sex. Although it is one of the most common cancers in women, affecting 1 woman in 80 with 2000 women dying every year, it is one of the easiest to diagnose, treat and cure if it detected early enough.

Ovarian cancer causes the deaths of up to 4,000 women every year, although it is rare in women under the age of 40. It is caused when abnormal tissue develops in the ovary and is sometimes related to ovarian cysts. It is very difficult to detect in its early stages because the ovaries are buried in the abdominal cavity. Any swelling is often not noticed until the disease is advanced; it is at this stage that there may be other symptoms including lower abdominal pain, weight loss and general ill-health.

Vaginal Cancer is extremely rare. The vagina connects the cervix with the vulva (the folds of skin around the opening to the vagina). There are two types of cancer of the vagina: squamous cell cancer (squamous carcinoma) and adenocarcinoma. Squamous carcinoma is usually found in women between the ages of 60 and 80. Adenocarcinoma is more often found in women between the ages of 12 and 30.

Cancer of the Vulva occurs in the outer part of a woman's vagina. Most women with cancer of the vulva are over age 50. However, it is becoming more common in women under age

40. Women who have constant itching, changes in the color and the way the vulva looks should discuss these symptoms with their doctor. A doctor should also be consulted if there is bleeding or discharge not related to menstruation (periods), severe burning/itching or pain in the vulva, or if the skin of the vulva looks white and feels rough.

Endometriosis has no agreed theory that explains why it occurs; however there are claims that more that one million women suffer from it in the UK and the Endometriosis Society suggests that an average length of time to make a diagnosis is about seven years.

The OXEGENE (Oxford Endometriosis Study) study is currently taking place at the Nuffield Department of Obstetrics and Gynaecology at the University of Oxford in the UK to determine if there is a genetic reason for endometriosis. This international study involves women who have another member of their immediate family who also have the condition.   For more information you can visit their web pages at: *http://www.medicine.ox.ac.uk/ndog/oxegene/oxegene.htm*

Endometriosis occurs when the cells of the endometrium (lining of the uterus) are found in other parts of the body. In the same way that the lining of the uterus swells and sheds each month as a period; these growths also swell and bleed, but as they are embedded in tissue, the blood cannot escape and so it forms blood blisters that will in turn irritate and scar the surrounding tissue which will then form a fibrous cyst around the blister. This can also result in scarring on the ovaries, fallopian tubes and uterus which may then lead to infertility as they can make transfer of an ovum (egg) from the ovary to the fallopian tube very difficult. They can also stop passage of an egg down the fallopian tube to the uterus. Occasionally when the scarring is very bad, it can stick to the wall of the abdominal cavity and other organs which will be painful when it tears away and leave scars.

It is believed to be caused by a "retrograde menstruation" where fragments of the lining are shed backwards rather than through the vagina. Women may suffer no symptoms at all or they may be great pain when they have a period or during sex, and periods may be very heavy. Initial treatment will be with hormone drugs that either reduce or stop the periods altogether and which allow the blisters to heal. However if the ovaries are affected then removal may be necessary.

Fibroids A fibroid is a benign tumor of the uterus and it will often appear either within the muscular wall of the uterus or on the outside of the wall. It is thought that around 30% of all hysterectomies performed in the United States are due to fibroids and it is estimated that between 25-35% of all women will have fibroids of varying sizes.

It is not known what causes fibroids, although it is known that they are related to the production of oestrogen. However, there are no clear studies showing that women who have fibroids have higher than average levels of oestrogen. It is known that, as with endometriosis, they will usually shrink following the menopause.

The rate at which they grow depends on the individual woman. They can range between very small to the size of a melon and the size may bear no relation to the severity of the symptoms experienced. Women may also experience problems with the bladder if the fibroid presses on it. Finally they may also find that sex is painful.

Fibroids may also interfere with conception if they protrude into the uterus. They may also be a cause of premature births if they are taking up too much room within the uterus. Both of these instances only happen rarely.

The Center for Uterine Fibroids based at the Brigham and Women's Hospital in Boston, Massachusetts has been conducting a study to determine if there is a genetic link to fibroids. The study is due to end in mid 2005.

Heavy Vaginal Bleeding Regular bleeding as it is known today is a relatively new experience for women. In the last one hundred years the number of periods experienced by women across their lifetime has increased from an average of 40 to 400.

Heavy vaginal bleeding usually refers to heavy periods (Menorrhagia), although it can also mean bleeding between periods and/or periods lasting longer than a week. The amount of blood that you lose will depend on your own hormone levels through your cycle. Bleeding differs between women and the perception of what is a heavy bleed is often very different; what is heavy for one woman may be fairly light for another. The average period lasts for five days and a woman can expect to lose about two tablespoons of blood during that time, although it does look a lot more.

A heavy period is defined by the Medical Profession as one that has a total blood loss of more than 80ml which is equivalent to half a cupful of liquid. Other definitions may include periods that last longer that seven days, one where large clots of blood are passed or if flooding occurs. It can be a symptom of other conditions, such as endometriosis, fibroids or pelvic inflammatory disease and it is possible that having a coil fitted for contraceptive purposes can make periods heavier and/or more painful. They can be caused by high levels of the female sex hormones or by an imbalance in the prostaglandins which are a naturally occurring substance in the body. According to the RCOG (Royal College of Obstetricians and Gynaecologists) approximately one in 20 women report heavy blood loss.

There is also a danger of developing anaemia due to iron deficiency so it is important to make sure that you keep to a well balanced diet. You may find that your daily life is also affected because of the flooding and/or pain.   Treatment with hormones or the contraceptive pill and iron tablets may be tried and you may also be offered a "trans-cervical re-section" of the lining of the uterus, where the lining of the uterus is taken away.

According to Herbert Goldfarb, 70% of women who experience problems with their periods are at the extremes of their menstrual life, that is they are just beginning or they are reaching the menopause. He also states that 70% of them are also not ovulating and that this can be the most common cause of heavy bleeding. This lack of ovulation results in a woman producing no progesterone which means that the oestrogen production enables the lining of the uterus to carry on growing without stopping. When the lining eventually begins to break down, the resultant blood loss is extremely heavy.

In the US, the MS (Medicine or Surgery) Study is a nationwide research study being conducted in four American cities to understand how well commonly used treatments work for women with abnormal uterine bleeding.

Pelvic inflammatory disease or salpingitis occurs when microbes get into the uterus causing an infection which can then spread to the fallopian tubes, ovaries and surrounding tissues. It is often, but not always, introduced during sex (through sexually transmitted disease's such as gonorrhea or chlamydia).

It is also possible that it may also occur following abdominal surgery. Other common causes include childbirth and associated operations. With a mild attack of Pelvic Inflammatory Disease a woman runs a 3% chance of having a blocked fallopian tube; when the number of bad attacks is three or more then her chance increases to 75%.

If no treatment is undertaken then there is the potential for it to spread further into the reproductive system and it can eventually cause fertility problems.

Following treatment, if symptoms recur then it may be necessary to have a laparoscopy (a small incision is made in the abdomen and a camera is inserted into the uterus) in hospital to check on the diagnosis.

Prolapse is a term used to cover a variety of conditions that may or may not affect a woman's need for a hysterectomy. They are referred to by the wider term of 'genital prolapse' which includes several conditions. These can occur separately or together and they may occur to differing degrees. These include uterine prolapse (dropped uterus), vaginal prolapse, cystocele (dropped bladder), rectocele (dropped rectum), and enterocele (hernia of the small intestine into the space between the rectum and vagina).

Uterine prolapse or dropped uterus is a condition in which the uterus drops downward in the pelvis below its normal position. The uterus may drop slightly and remain above the vagina or it may drop further so that the cervix or lower portion of the uterus reaches into the vagina. In its worst form, the cervix or even the entire uterus will protrude out of the vagina.

All prolapses occur when the muscles and ligaments holding these organs to the bones of the pelvis become weak. Stretching and slackening is a natural result of childbirth and also takes place as you get older. When the muscles and ligaments no longer work the uterus and vagina will sag down and a bulge of the bladder or rectum may occur in the front or back wall of the vagina. It can also occur due to a thinning of the muscles at the time of the menopause which, in turn, is caused by a drop in the female sex hormones. Another common cause of prolapse is obesity which can add additional stresses to an already weak system of support with the extra weight pressing on the bladder.

Occasionally prolapse may occur if there is an inherited weakness of the pelvic floor muscles. The most common types of delivery to cause problems with prolapse are those that are protracted, are for large babies or use forceps or a vacuum extraction. Occasionally heavy lifting, chronic coughing or constipation can also be cited as reasons for a later prolapse of other organs in the abdominal region.

Certain types of prolapse can lead to varying levels or severity of urinary incontinence. The different types of incontinence include:

- Stress incontinence where urine is leaked when a woman coughs, sneezes or laughs for instance.
- Urge incontinence where a woman feels a need to go to the toilet more frequently than necessary
- Overflow incontinence where the bladder fills and is not emptied properly
- Total incontinence where there is a constant loss of urine.

Emergencies such as rupture or puncture of the uterus during other surgery and problems at childbirth may lead to uncontrollable bleeding which may be impossible to stop. In these cases hysterectomy is a life saver.

HOW MIGHT A HYSTERECTOMY AFFECT YOU?

You do need to be absolutely sure that you know what the operation will mean for your long term future. This may result in preferring to live with your condition if, for instance, you would like to have children at a later stage. How you feel after having had a hysterectomy will depend a great deal on your personal circumstances and why the operation became necessary in the first place.

Physically, there are a number of issues that are common to all women having a hysterectomy. You will not have any more periods and you will not be able to have any more children. If you have had your ovaries removed you will go through the menopause, regardless of your age (unless you have already done so). The menopause is not related to age, it is related to the production of the female sex hormone, oestrogen. If your ovaries are removed, your GP and/or surgeon will discuss Hormone Replacement Therapy with you to help you deal with the effects of the menopause. If you have not had your ovaries removed and you have not gone through the menopause before your operation, there is up to a 50% chance that you will also go through the menopause within two to five years of having the operation.

Immediately following the operation you will spend some time in hospital recovering. The length of time will depend on the type of operation you have had. You will be encouraged to get out of bed as soon as possible. This will help your recovery and will improve your circulation to avoid the danger of blood clots forming. You may also experience painful wind that will gradually fade over a few days.

Once at home you will be advised not to be too active for at least six weeks; this is to give time for the muscles and tissues in the abdomen to heal. There may be gentle exercises that your GP or surgeon may suggest and you will probably be encouraged to walk (slowly) a little every day. Try to increase the length of time that you go out for on a daily basis, without pushing yourself too hard. You should be aware that it can take a long time to recover from this type of surgery, even up to twelve months. Generally however, after six - eight weeks you should be able to take on some lighter household tasks and even to return to work part-time. However, this will depend on the type of work that you do.

Sexually, you may resume intercourse after about six weeks. However you may find that it is different in some ways. This will depend again on why you had your hysterectomy and the type of operation you have had.

Although many women report that their sex life improves following a hysterectomy, as they are not experiencing pain any longer, others report that they have different types or intensities of orgasm. This may be due to the removal of the contractual muscles (the uterus and cervix) as it is not just the clitoris that is involved in creating an orgasm. Therefore, orgasm may be less intense when they have been removed.

It is also possible that a deficiency of the hormone, oestrogen, also affects a woman's sexuality. It is well documented that one of the symptoms of the menopause is dryness of the vagina. We are now aware, as well, that the hormone, testosterone, also plays a part in sexuality. The removal of both of these hormones may contribute to a lack of sexual interest, frequency and orgasm. These are symptoms that may be alleviated by the use of Hormone Replacement Therapy.

Emotionally you may find that you have low mood following your operation. This may be due to having gone through major surgery which is traumatic in itself. However, you may also be dealing with the shock of finding that you had a serious illness as well and some women report a feeling of loss as they are aware that they can no longer have children or that they feel they are no longer "womanly".

It has also been suggested that some of these feelings may be due to the onset of the menopause as well as the lack of testosterone that occurs when the ovaries are removed or fail. If you have had your ovaries removed or are suffering from some other menopausal symptoms you may benefit from talking to your GP about Hormone Replacement Therapy.

It often helps to talk about your experiences with other people in the same position as yourself. There may be a menopause or well-woman clinic at your hospital, surgery or in the nearest large town. Alternatively, you could try contacting one of the many support organisations that are available for information and support, and those listed at the back of this book. You can also read the discussion pages of The Hysterectomy Association web site where other women record their experiences and ask questions.

Of course many women find that they feel wonderful, because they are free of the heavy bleeding and/or the pain that has dogged them for so long. It can be wonderfully invigorating not to be tied to tampons and pads any longer. Try to remember that all women are different and each will react to the operation differently. Whatever feelings you experience they are unique to you and are your own way of dealing with a hysterectomy.

ALTERNATIVES TO HYSTERECTOMY

Hysterectomy is a serious operation causing the uterus and other organs to be permanently removed. There may be a case then for trying to prevent this radical step if at all possible. A number of alternative treatments for the various gynaecological conditions, mostly surgical, have been developed.

Not all alternatives will be appropriate for all women or even available in all parts of the UK, and if women are interested in any of the alternatives discussed they should contact their doctor or gynaecologist for a discussion about the viability in their particular case.

Uterine Arterial Embolisation can be used to remove fibroids that are growing in the uterus or uterine wall. The proponents of the technique believe that it may involve the lowest risk of surgery as well as the briefest recovery time.

The procedure is carried out by an Interventional Radiologist and involves a catheter being inserted into the uterus together with the injection of synthetic particles into the blood vessel supplying the fibroid. The intention is that the particles will block the flow of blood to the fibroid and once cut off this will then cause the fibroid to shrink and thus alleviate the pain, bleeding and other symptoms associated with it. It has also been used to reduce the size of fibroids so that less radical surgery can be carried out. The surgery is usually carried out under local anaesthetic and therefore carries fewer risks.

Although NICE (the National Institute for Clinical Effectiveness) have given their consent to this procedure they have indicated that there are a number of side effects that might occur. These may include severe pain, high temperature, haematoma, nausea and sickness, infection, blockage to the bowel, passing the fibroid out of the body through the vagina and cramping following the surgery. However, the majority of women will be back to normal within a few days. If you have been offered this type of surgery it would be worth discussing the risk of side effects with your GP and/or consultant.

Surgical Endometrial Ablation and Resection has been around for about 10 years and has been used in the treatment of heavy bleeding as well as the removal of fibroids and polyps. Various studies have shown a success rate of around 85% in reducing or eliminating bleeding. However, this procedure does cause infertility as it involves the removal of the uterus lining (the endometrium). One of the advantages of the technique is that it can be performed under local anaesthetic, takes about an hour and most women are able to resume normal activities in two to five days.

Myomectomy is the surgical removal of fibroids from the uterus leaving the uterus intact. There are a number of alternative ways to perform the surgery. The most common is via an abdominal incision on the bikini line and is most appropriate where the fibroids are large, numerous or in many different locations. Whether it can be performed or not will be dependent on where the fibroids are located.

A myomectomy can also be performed vaginally through the cervix and is best suited to those fibroids that are small, on the inside of the uterine wall and which usually have a stalk. This procedure may be performed under local anaesthetic after the cervix has been enlarged overnight. It is minimally invasive.

Laparoscopic and hysteroscopic myomectomies are also minimally invasive but are more difficult to perform. They require the use of a laparoscope (small camera) and small abdominal incision. Gas is used in the abdomen to move the various organs out of the way so that the surgeon can see clearly. It is a procedure best suited to small and superficial fibroids. In some cases a laser can be used with the hysteroscope to remove fibroids, although this is not routinely available in the UK due to the high cost of equipment.

Myoma Coagulation or Myolysis involves the use of intense heat or lasers via needles that will kill off the fibroid and its blood supply. The heat is used to cut, cauterise and vaporise the blood vessel and tissue. It is very minimally invasive as it does not require an incision for the laparoscope to pass into the abdomen. The laparoscope is used via the vagina and cervix. This is probably not a preferred treatment for women that wish to have children, as there is, currently, little research evidence to show that pregnancy is completed satisfactory following the procedure and it is possible that scar tissue may form and interfere with conception.

Laser and Thermal Balloon Ablation are promising new procedures in the treatment of heavy bleeding. Thermal balloon ablation is a second generation endometrial ablation technique and involves the insertion of a balloon filled with hot water into the uterus which removes the endometrium from the uterus. It is used to treat heavy bleeding in some women. It has also recently been the subject of a review by NICE (The National Institute of Clinical Excellence) to determine whether it is an appropriate treatment for use on NHS patients. NICE have now said that it is an appropriate treatment if their guidelines are followed.

During treatment a small balloon is inserted via a catheter through the vagina into the uterus. The balloon is then filled with fluid and the fluid is heated to 87°C. This pressure and temperature is maintained for around eight minutes which should be enough to remove the endometrial lining of the uterus.

Laser surgery is another form of endometrial ablation and is a simple procedure in which the doctor looks through a hysteroscope (a small telescope inserted into the abdomen) and removes the uterine lining. The procedure is very rapid and will enable a patient to leave hospital within a few hours in most cases. There is frequently a vaginal discharge for several days but significant problems with recovery such as pain, infection, or bleeding seem to be rare. However, the cost of the equipment used in this type of treatment means that it is not very widely available.

One other consideration to bear in mind is that removal of the lining of the uterus, the endometrium, will mean that it is not possible to have children in the future.

Microwave Endometrial Ablation (MEA) has recently been recommended by NICE (The National Institute for Clinical Excellence) as an appropriate treatment for some women who suffer from heavy bleeding, provided that appropriate protocols for patient selection, training and operation techniques are followed. However, MEA is not necessarily a replacement for hysterectomy as there may be some cases where it is not a suitable treatment.

MEA uses heat from a microwave probe to remove or reduce the thickness of the lining of the uterus. Almost every one of 600 women in the clinical trial, who had MEA treatment reported that their blood loss during a period was significantly reduced. Research evidence has indicated that blood loss was completely stopped in around 62% of cases. About 70% of the cases treated also found that their period pain disappeared or reduced significantly.

Once the probe has been inserted into the uterus it is moved around from side to side and a temperature of 75 to 80°C is maintained. Patients are admitted as day cases as opposed to in-patient cases. The research has also shown that the average length of time that it takes to perform the surgery is 11-15 minutes. After the surgery patients are expected to take between two to four days to recover.

Most women with endometriosis are treated with pain relief and hormones. Women who don't respond may be offered minimally invasive surgery to remove or vaporise the endometrial deposits, most commonly by cauterization or laser through a laparoscope. Women with very severe symptoms may be offered more radical treatment by hysterectomy and removal of the ovaries.

Laparoscopic helium plasma coagulation of endometriosis is a minimally invasive procedure used to vaporise endometrial deposits. Using a laparoscope, an ionised beam of helium gas is directed at endometrial deposits to destroy them. However, it is probably best for very superficial endometriosis as studies have identified damage to deeper tissue and other organs as a potential risk. It is also important that the surgeons have specialist surgical training. There is little clinical research or evidence to be able to comment on how effective this type of treatment is and whether it will be commonly available in the near future.

Drug and other treatments There are a variety of alternative drug treatments, for some of the conditions that may lead to a hysterectomy. These include:

- A low dose contraceptive pill can reduce bleeding in half of the women who try it.
- Tranexamic acid, which is used to promote blood clotting, can cut bleeding in 60% of cases, although pain is not reduced.
- Mefanamic acid, an inflammatory drug can reduce bleeding by 20% and ease period pain. But possible side effects include nausea, vomiting and kidney problems. These drug treatments will not affect your long-term fertility.
- A common treatment for endometriosis is Danol, a drug which induces a false menopause. It can be effective for many women, but does have side effects related to the menopause. These can include hot flushes and night sweats, as well as facial hair growth. Other side effects include nausea, dizziness, rash, backache, muscle spasm and fluid retention.

The Mirena Intrauterine System (IUS) or coil can also reduce heavy bleeding. It's fitted by a GP and left in place within the uterus. After three months use the average blood loss is expected to reduce by 85% and after 12 months the flow can be reduced by up to 97%. About one third of women will have no periods at all, as the progesterone in the IUS prevents the lining of the uterus from building up.

One study looked at 54 women with heavy periods who were awaiting a hysterectomy. After being fitted with the Mirena IUS, around 70% were taken off the waiting list because they were so happy with the treatment.

However, possible side effects include headache, water retention and breast tenderness. Pregnancy is rare, but if it does occur it is advisable to remove the contraceptive as soon as possible to reduce the risk of bleeding, infection or miscarriage.

RECOVERING AFTER HYSTERECTOMY

It is normal during the first 24-36 hours after surgery to feel many aches and pains all over your body. It is usual to experience backache, shoulder pain and a stiff neck as well as abdominal pain.

You may find you are attached to a PCA (Patient Controlled Analgesia). This is usually morphine and it means you will be in control of your own pain medication.

During your operation, you may well have been catheterised. It means that straight after the operation when you are at your most uncomfortable you do not have to worry about going to a toilet to pass urine. This will be simply passed into a bag at your side and emptied regularly by the nurses. It will be removed after the first 24 hours and is painless.

Drink plenty of water, to replace that lost through the anaesthetic and operation. You will probably be attached to a saline drip to help you re-hydrate as well.

You may have some slight vaginal bleeding; this is normal and should soon clear up. A mild and gentle laxative can help you to open your bowels; this will make you feel more comfortable. You might also have some trapped wind and indigestion due to lack of movement; this can be relieved by medication and/or by gentle exercise.

Once you return home you must make sure that you are taking things easy. Your hospital physiotherapist can give some exercises to do to help you get back to full mobility.

As you shouldn't be lifting anything heavy, such as shopping, for a while it is important that you have a support network around to help out. If you live alone and this isn't possible ask your nurse for the details of a local support network that can help.

Gentle walking, a little further each day, will help to get your circulation working properly. It is normally around six weeks before patients think about a return to work, however this will depend on the type of work that you do. For instance if you have to do heavy lifting or very physical work it may take a lot longer to recover fully enough to return.

A little backache and discomfort in the abdomen are common for the first few weeks after surgery. If you have a browny discharge this should change to creamy white. You may also notice that the internal stitches are passed out of the body as well.

If you have any pain, pus, fresh blood or smelly discharge you should see your doctor as soon as possible.

THE RISKS ASSOCIATED WITH HYSTERECTOMY

For the majority of women a hysterectomy will a liberating experience and they will go on to lead perfectly normal lives, however for a very small number the reverse may be true and we have listed a number of the risks which may be related to having a hysterectomy:

- Irritable bowel syndrome which is stress related
- Stress incontinence or other urinary symptoms
- Damage to the urethra and bowel; this risk may be slightly increased if the cervix is removed due to its proximity to these organs
- Prolapse of the vagina
- Back pain
- Depression
- Loss of sexual feeling and function
- Post operative infection
- Haematoma (a collection of blood under the wound)
- Thrombosis (blood clot)
- Hysterectomy has also been known to trigger arthritis, but the reason for this is unknown.

Some other conditions may also re-occur, this might include, adhesions, pelvic inflammatory disease and endometriosis. These are probably because they are all triggered by oestrogen, which the body will continue to produce naturally if a woman retains her ovaries or if a woman takes HRT when her ovaries are removed.   If you experience any of these conditions you must seek the advice and help of your doctor.

THE MENOPAUSE

If you have your ovaries removed at the time of your hysterectomy then you will have an immediate menopause, regardless of your age (unless you have already gone through it). If you have a hysterectomy and your ovaries are left intact then you have up to a 50% chance of your ovaries failing within two to five years of your hysterectomy. This may be because the blood supply to the uterus has been cut off. Radiation treatment following hysterectomy for cancer may also cause the ovaries to fail early.

Even after a natural menopause the ovaries continue to play a part in a woman's health as they continue to produce a small amount of oestrogen and a more significant amount of testosterone for up to 12 years. Therefore there are indications that women having a hysterectomy may be offered testosterone therapy as well as oestrogen.

Menopausal Symptoms

Strictly speaking, the symptoms of the menopause are those that identify the time leading up to the final bleed. This is usually called the peri-menopause. However, a menopause following hysterectomy can be called a Surgical Menopause. Symptoms can be physical and/or emotional in nature. Some of the symptoms are described as *acute* and they will occur immediately there is a reduction in the production of oestrogen. They include hot flushes, night sweats, dry vagina, dry hair and skin, insomnia, bladder problems and moodiness. The remainder are described as *chronic* and take place over a longer period of time. These include breast changes and emotional problems.

All women that have a hysterectomy that removes their ovaries will begin to experience acute symptoms, as early as 24 hours following surgery. If you have had surgery that leaves your ovaries intact and you begin to experience some of the symptoms described below you should make an appointment to see your GP to have a simple blood test to measure the level of oestrogen in your blood.

Physical symptoms may include hot and cold flushes, sweating during the day and/or at night and palpitations, which are all known as vasomotor symptoms. The exact causes of the vasomotor symptoms are unknown but it is thought probable that the hypothalamus, which regulates body temperature, is affected by the decrease in oestrogen production and this in turn dilates the blood vessels which affects the sympathetic nervous system. It is thought that up to 80% of women will experience some of these symptoms.

Insomnia and headaches are secondary vasomotor symptoms and can occur as a result of night sweats which can result in loss of sleep.

Changes in the vagina include shortening and weakening of the skin, a lack of elasticity, diminishing blood supply to the skin, changes in the acidity levels and dryness due to the reduction in secretions from the mucous glands. All of these can lead to pain with sex and an increase in the risk of bleeding and infection. The bladder and urethra can also be affected as the linings become thin and weak and stress incontinence can occur as these organs atrophy. This increases the risk of infection and bleeding.

Breast changes occur as a direct result of the reduction in production of oestrogen. The breasts may become smaller and less elastic and the skin will become thinner and dryer.

The skin and hair become dryer and the elasticity of the skin reduces which increases the appearance of wrinkles. The changes in the skin are due to damaging effects on the connective tissue, collagen, when oestrogen production reduces.

Emotional symptoms are similar to those experienced with pre-menstrual syndrome and may include: mood swings, irritability, anxiety, poor concentration, poor memory, loss of energy and depression.

It cannot be confirmed at present whether these symptoms are caused by oestrogen deprivation or whether they are as a result of other physical symptoms, such as lack of sleep.

However, some sleep disorders are helped by hormone replacement therapy, so there does appear to be a link with oestrogen deficiency.

Menopause or Thyroid?

It has been suggested that women that are starting to experience menopausal symptoms, particularly if they are younger than the average age for menopause and have not had their ovaries removed, should have not only a blood oestrogen test, but should also have a test to check that their thyroid is still functioning properly. Many symptoms that are associated with a dysfunctional thyroid gland are similar to those of the menopause.

Oestrogen

Oestrogen is a powerful female sex hormone that regulates many aspects of our lives. Initially it makes girls develop into women at puberty by stimulating breast growth, laying down fatty deposits, thickening the vagina and causing it to secrete mucous. It affects how our skin looks, whether our bones are strong and healthy and it can protect us against heart disease. It also regulates our menstrual cycle. At the beginning of our cycle about 30 egg follicles will start to ripen and produce oestrogen. When levels of oestrogen in the blood are highest; the hypothalamus in the brain releases hormones that make a follicle release an egg. Therefore if you are not producing enough oestrogen you will not ovulate.

Oestrogen can also affect your mood and it is thought that pre-menstrual syndrome, post-natal depression and menopausal depression are caused by falling levels of oestrogen. Your exposure to oestrogen may also have an effect on your risk of developing breast cancer as it attaches itself to receptors in the breast on the surface of cells and stimulates them to divide in anticipation of producing milk; it is the unrestricted division of these cells that is thought to be implicated in breast cancer.

There is no 'standard' as far as the natural amounts of oestrogen produced are concerned. Women vary in their needs during their lifetime. When a woman has a hysterectomy that removes her ovaries, she will no longer produce oestrogen from them. She will continue to produce oestrogen in the adrenal gland and in fatty tissues but these are only very small amounts and are not enough to prevent menopausal symptoms or ensure long term health.

Oestrogen is the main component of Hormone Replacement Therapy that is taken by women who have had a hysterectomy. It can be taken in many different forms and although called natural, it is manufactured. The term "natural" is used because the hormones that are produced are identical to those produced by the human body.

Progesterone

Progesterone is produced by a woman's ovaries when she ovulates. It supports the life of the unborn child in the uterus, but it also helps the body in many other ways, whether a woman is pregnant or not. It balances the effects of oestrogen, which can be destructive if not kept in check.

During the first half of the menstrual cycle, oestrogen is the dominant hormone, helping to prepare the uterus for a fertilized egg by building up the lining of the uterus. During the second half of the menstrual cycle progesterone is the dominant hormone and ensures that a bleed occurs to remove the lining of the uterus if it is not needed to support a foetus. It also prevents any further ovulation taking place, closes the cervix and makes the vaginal mucus acidic to kill any remaining sperm.

For women who have had a hysterectomy, it is not normally considered necessary to supplement with progesterone as there is no uterine lining to shed.

Testosterone

Testosterone is a male hormone but women still produce small amounts. Testosterone is produced by the ovaries and helps to regulate sex drive (libido), energy and mental state. Following a natural menopause testosterone will continue to be produced by the ovaries for approximately twelve years; therefore a woman who has a surgical menopause that removes her ovaries will no longer produce testosterone and this may be responsible for a reduced libido, depression and a lack of energy following surgery. Testosterone may have a role to play in conserving bone mass after menopause and may be more suitable for women that are unable to take oestrogen supplements who also have an increased risk of osteoporosis.

However testosterone should not be taken orally, in the form of tablets as it can damage the liver. The usual form of administration is by implant or by injection at regular intervals.

Osteoporosis

Osteoporosis is defined as "the wasting away of bone" and the term literally means "porous bones". It is often called the silent epidemic as many people can be unaware of its start and the first indication of the disease can be falling and breaking a bone. It is one of the biggest health risks following the menopause.

It has been considered a natural part of ageing although with treatment it is largely preventable. Osteoporosis is most common in the elderly and in post-menopausal women. It is caused by the loss of calcium from the bones. Bones continue to grow and develop throughout childhood and adolescence and the bones are at their most dense around the age of 30. After this age, bone density gradually diminishes.

Risk Factors for Osteoporosis

Oestrogen deficiency has been identified as one of the most important factors in the development of osteoporosis for women. Women undergoing hysterectomy before they would normally go through the menopause are more likely to develop osteoporosis than those in the same age group who go through the menopause naturally. Oestrogen deficiency occurs after the onset of the menopause. However, although oestrogen deficiency is a major factor there are others to take into account. These include:

- race, if you are white or Asian you are slightly more at risk
- build, if you are fine boned you will have a higher risk
- smoking
- being underweight
- diet consistently low in calcium and high in phosphates
- excessive alcohol and caffeine intake
- family history of osteoporosis
- lack of exercise
- use of cortisone-like drugs
- vitamin D deficiency
- being a woman; it is estimated to be six to eight times more common in women than in men, as women have a lower bone mass to start with

Prevention

It has been recommended that all women have a bone mineral density (BMD) test before they undergo a hysterectomy. This will determine how strong the bones are to start with and will provide a point of reference for later on. After the menopause, if you do not wish to take Hormone Replacement Therapy, it would be advisable to have regular BMD tests to ensure your continued health.

Regular blood tests to determine your levels of oestrogen are also recommended, particularly if you have a hysterectomy that leaves your ovaries intact. Your GP or gynaecologist should be able to arrange both of these procedures for you.

The most common way to prevent osteoporosis due to low oestrogen levels is to boost the levels of oestrogen with Hormone Replacement Therapy. Hormone Replacement Therapy (HRT) puts oestrogen back into the body. HRT has been shown to retard, stop and even reverse bone loss after the menopause.

Exercise is also highly recommended as this helps to strengthen bones and keep them strong. However, the type of exercise is very important; it should be regular and it should be weight bearing. Weight bearing exercises include any type of exercise that involves upright movement so that pressure is exerted through the spine, pelvis and legs and includes walking, jogging, aerobics and yoga.

Your diet is also particularly important as it should contain high levels of calcium and vitamin D (Vitamin D can be obtained from being out in the sunshine) and should be low in fat and high in fibre.

However, recent guidelines published by the Medicines and Healthcare Products Regulatory Agency (MHRA) have recommended that GP's do not use HRT as an initial treatment for osteoporosis. They have recommended that it is a suitable treatment for women who can't take any other treatment for osteoporosis.

Heart Disease

Heart Disease is the biggest single cause of death in the UK in post-menopausal women. Up to the time of the menopause, women appear to have a natural immunity to heart disease unlike their male counterparts. However, after the age of menopause the incidence gradually increases to come into line with men at around the age of 75. It is believed that it is the production of oestrogen that provides this natural immunity. Therefore, pre-menopausal women who have a hysterectomy may have up to three times the risk of coronary heart disease and this may even be the case even when the ovaries are left intact.

We can also assume that if a woman has a hysterectomy and consequently goes through the menopause early, the age at which she comes into line with male incidence of heart disease will be correspondingly lower.

Risk Factors

Particularly at risk are the following groups:

- smokers
- people that are overweight
- families with a history of heart disease
- women with high levels of cholesterol before the operation
- women that do not take regular exercise.

Prevention

In addition to HRT, a healthy diet and regular exercise will do much to mitigate the causes of heart disease in later life. In addition to helping prevent heart disease, a healthier diet and exercise will also help to prevent blood clots, reduce your cholesterol levels and improve your metabolism; all things which also help to reduce the risk of heart disease.

However, recent research evidence has been conflicting in its approach to the appropriateness of HRT as a preventive medicine against heart disease. One study carried out by the Women's Health Initiative has suggested that HRT provides no visible benefits in preventing heart disease, whilst another carried out at the Hammersmith NHS Trust in London have shown that it is effective in preventing heart disease. The advice being given by the British Heart Foundation is that women should discuss their options with their GP, taking into account, the age, whether they have had an early or surgical menopause and other health related factors. They will then be able to make an informed decision about what is appropriate for them.

HORMONE REPLACEMENT THERAPY

HRT is the substitution of naturally occurring hormones in the human body with those that are manufactured. In the case of women that have had a hysterectomy we are talking about oestrogen and possibly testosterone replacement therapies. When a woman has had a hysterectomy that removes her ovaries she will no longer produce oestrogen from her ovaries although she will continue to produce small amounts of oestrogen from the adrenal glands and fatty tissues. However, this will not be enough to counteract the possible effects of oestrogen deficiency that we see begin with menopausal symptoms.

There are many things that women need to consider when they are faced with a surgical menopause and one of the major issues is whether or not to take HRT. It can be beneficial in alleviating the symptoms of the menopause. Women should also consider the fact that they will be longer without the female sex hormones than their age related peers and that some of the natural protections that are offered by the sex hormones are lost. These include protection against Heart Disease and Osteoporosis.

Some early studies have also indicated that oestrogen supplementation in the form of HRT may also lessen the risk of developing Alzheimer's disease, although this must be the subject of future research projects.

There seems to be some agreement that women who have an early menopause through surgery should take HRT at least until the age that they would naturally have gone through the menopause. This is so that they reduce the risk of suffering from age related conditions like osteoporosis and heart disease earlier than they would have done. Women naturally produce oestrogen up to the age of the menopause and it would appear to be sensible to replace what would be produced naturally.

What a woman decides to do after the age of 50ish will be determined by looking at the same factors that affect all women and will again be a matter of choice. At the very least women who still have ovaries after surgery should be having regular blood tests to check the amount of oestrogen they are producing so that they can make an informed choice.

There seems to be little argument that HRT taken for up to five years *after a natural menopause* does not adversely affect the body and there seems to be some evidence that women who do develop breast cancer have a better prognosis if they have taken HRT than if they had not, although this may of course be related to the type of cancer that they have.

Women should, however, take into account a number of factors when considering whether to take HRT or not.

In favour of taking HRT are:

- family history of osteoporosis
- high risk category related to osteoporosis
- family history of heart disease
- high risk category related to heart disease
- fear of Alzheimer's disease
- Severe menopause symptoms

You may also consider *not* taking HRT for the following reasons:

- history of breast cancer
- family history of breast cancer
- high risk category related to breast cancer
- history of thrombosis
- family history of thrombosis
- high risk category of thrombosis

Prior to a undergoing a hysterectomy it may be beneficial to have a blood oestrogen test so that there is some indication of your normal oestrogen levels. These can then be used as comparisons later on.

Types of Hormone Replacement Therapy

Not all types of HRT will suit all women and it is important to work with your GP to find the most suitable form of treatment for your own particular circumstances.

Tablets are the most common way to administer HRT and must be taken every day. As the tablets pass through the liver, higher doses of oestrogen need to be used in them, as about 30% of it is made inactive by the liver.

Patches are used on clean dry skin and placed on the buttocks or the lower abdomen. They are applied every three to four days and have few side effects other than skin irritation which can be lessened by using talcum powder on the skin first. They also have a habit of falling off when they get wet or in hot weather and can be embarrassing to use. As the oestrogen is not passing through the liver though, much smaller doses can be used to achieve the same hormonal effects.

Implants of oestrogen are placed underneath the skin in the area of the abdomen. The implant is small, about the size of an apple pip and it is inserted under local anaesthetic. This implant can last for up to six months and you will know when you need to have another one because you will begin to experience some menopausal symptoms, such as hot flushes and night sweats. The implant has advantages over other forms of administration as it avoids the liver and does not cause skin irritation as patches can. Because the oestrogen is not passing through the liver, the amount of oestrogen in the implant can be reduced.

However, the implant is not without its own possible side effect. A small number of implant users experience a syndrome called tachyphylaxis, which means that the dosage needs to be increased to obtain the same effect even though the levels of blood oestrogen are high enough. This usually happens when a new implant is inserted before the last one has finished completely. This side effect has led to claims that HRT is addictive however, by careful monitoring a GP can allow patients to continue to use other forms of HRT to allow the body to settle down.

Creams, Gels and Pessaries. Oestrogen Gel has recently been released in the UK although it has been used in Europe for some time, Oestrogen cream has been used for some time. The cream or gel is rubbed onto the skin of the upper arm or inner thigh every day, making sure it is fully absorbed. The irritation that may be experienced with patches is avoided with the creams and gels. Again smaller doses can be administered as the oestrogen is not passing through the liver first. Pessaries are inserted high into the vagina and absorbed through the skin of the vagina into the blood stream as with creams and gels. Some women have reported an increase in libido when using pessaries and they do help to prevent vaginal dryness.

Side Effects of HRT

The following have been listed as side effects of HRT; you may or may not experience any or all of them with different brands:

- Gastro-Intestinal upsets
- Nausea and vomiting
- Weight gain
- Breast tenderness and enlargement
- Headaches and migraine
- Dizziness
- Impaired liver function
- Exacerbation of varicose veins
- Increased blood pressure
- Thrombosis
- Breast cancer

If you are taking HRT and experience any of these symptoms you should see your doctor to have appropriate tests and if necessary a change or reduction in the HRT prescribed.

Thrombosis

Deep Vein Thrombosis (DVT) refers to blood clots that can

partially or completely block a blood vessel. The condition occurs most frequently in the legs but it can occur almost anywhere from the lower abdomen down. Deep vein thrombosis is fairly rare and affects about 1 person in 1700. People who are particularly susceptible are the elderly, those that are overweight and those who have a condition called polycythaemia (inability to control the rise in numbers of red blood cells). Deep vein thrombosis can cause pulmonary embolism which is potentially fatal. A pulmonary embolism happens when pieces of a blood clot break away and become lodged in an artery in the lungs thus reducing the amount of oxygenated blood going to the heart.

The incidence of deep vein thrombosis appears to increase by up to four times in HRT users and the risk seems to be higher when treatment is first started and reduces significantly with long term use. In a woman that is categorised as low risk, this may mean an increase of 1 in 5000. Any woman that already has a history of deep vein thrombosis or pulmonary embolism should avoid taking HRT, unless the thrombosis was as a result of surgery, accident, pregnancy or childbirth in which case there should not be an increased risk.

Breast Cancer

Perhaps the publics' most significant concern about Hormone Replacement Therapy (HRT) is that of a possible increased risk of breast cancer. Breast cancer is an oestrogen dependent cancer and accounts for approximately 25% of all female cancers that occur, therefore any woman who has an early menopause and does not take any oestrogen supplementation will actually reduce her risk of developing breast cancer in later life.

Currently about one woman in thirteen will develop breast cancer before the age of 75 and if there is a family history (sister or mother with the disease) the risk is increased to one in eight. Much of the initial data about the link with breast cancer and oestrogen supplementation has been taken from trials and studies based around the contraceptive pill. To date there have been over forty studies looking at the link between HRT and breast cancer and there has been no agreement about the results. It is also important to remember that most of the studies have also taken place on women that have gone through the menopause naturally rather than surgically. How much this may affect the outcome is unfortunately not known.

However, analysis of the studies estimates that there is no increase in risk when HRT is taken for up to five years. Women under 45*ish* who have a hysterectomy that removes their ovaries would naturally produce oestrogen if they hadn't been removed and in this case HRT may simply be replacing what they would normally produce.

Other risk factors associated with breast cancer include:

- previous history of oestrogen dependent cancers
- family history of cancer
- starting menstruation before the age of eleven
- not having a child or having your first child after the age of 30
- being overweight
- women who have diets high in fat and low in fibre also have a higher levels of oestrogen in the blood

The Million Women Study is a national study of how HRT affects women's health and involves around one million UK women aged 50 and over. It is a collaborative project between Cancer Research UK and the National Health Service. Initial findings have confirmed many of the other studies, showing that use of HRT can increase the risk of breast cancer. However, the risk is greatest for those women taking a combined oestrogen and progesterone HRT. Those taking oestrogen only, the majority will be women who have had a hysterectomy, are at less of a risk. You can find out more information from the web site at: *http://www.millionwomenstudy.org.uk/*

In 2003, the Medicine and Healthcare products Regulatory Agency produced the following guidance concerning use of Hormone Replacement Therapy.

- For short term treatment of menopausal symptoms the balance of risks and benefits is favourable. HRT therefore remains a suitable treatment option.

- HRT should however, only be used as a treatment to prevent osteoporosis by those who aren't able to take other osteoporosis treatments or for those where other treatment has been unsuccessful.
- There is no need to change your HRT if you have experienced an early menopause and are not yet 50 years old. However, treatment should be reviewed regularly.

ALTERNATIVES TO HORMONE REPLACEMENT THERAPY

Preventing Osteoporosis

Women can help to protect themselves against osteoporosis by taking HRT; however there may be some women who do not want to/can't, take it. They may be in a high risk category for Breast Cancer or Thrombosis. Or they may just not like taking drugs. However, before beginning any form of treatment, it is recommended that you discuss the options with your doctor and/or health practitioner.

Calcium is vitally important in the health of the bones and extra calcium after the menopause may help to reduce the loss of bone that occurs. It is as important to get adequate amounts of Vitamin D as this is used by the body as a bone strengthener and allows the body to absorb calcium effectively. Vitamin D is usually made naturally by the body when it is exposed to sunlight and it can also be found in fish, egg yolks and cereals. However those that find it difficult to get out in to the sun may find that taking supplements helps. You need to be taking at least 1,000mg of calcium per day. There are many foods that are very rich in calcium although those that are non dairy are less easily absorbed by the body than the calcium that you get from milk, fish (canned such as sardines and pilchard), hard cheeses (such as cheddar) and yoghurt. If you are a vegan you should be able to supplement your diet effectively with regular brazil nuts, almonds, green leafy vegetables, dried fruit, fortified soya milk, cereals and bread, although these are less easily absorbed.

Preventing Heart Disease

Diseases of the heart and strokes are the most common causes of death amongst post-menopausal women in the UK. In 1987 in England and Wales approximately 65,000 women died from heart disease and 45,000 from stoke. Compare this with the 18,000 deaths from breast cancer and you will put the risk into perspective. It is essential then that if you are unable or unwilling to take HRT that you reduce any risks by stopping smoking, reducing your weight, and taking exercise. Taking care with your diet is also important and there is some evidence that increasing your calcium intake can help to lower blood pressure. You can use semi or skimmed milk, low fat yoghurts and cheeses and increase other sources of plant calcium's from nuts, bread, cereals and leafy green vegetables.

The vitamins A, C and E are known as the anti-oxidant vitamins and play a key role in helping to keep your heart healthy. They help to reduce damage to the blood vessels by free radicals. Vitamin E also reduces damage to the good LDL (lower density lipoprotein) cholesterol.

Natural Plant Oestrogen's

There are over 300 plants that have oestrogen's in them and if they are consumed regularly enough they can have a mild effect on women. The most potent of the plant oestrogen's is Coumestrol even though it is about 200 times weaker than human oestrogen. Because the plant oestrogen's have such a mild effect the side effects found with conventional HRT should be avoided. Coumestrol can be found in alfalfa and red clover and can be taken either as tea or sprouted. The seeds must be obtained from a reputable herbalist or health food shop.

Other good sources of natural oestrogens are Soya beans, soybean sprouts and crushed linseeds. To vary the diet try to include good helpings of apples, beets, cabbage, carrots, chick peas, cucumbers, green beans, oats, olives, parsley, potatoes, rhubarb, rice, sesame seeds and sunflower seeds. There are many others but those on this list should be readily available from high street shops.

Other Dietary Supplements

Supplements are useful for women going through the menopause and can help protect against some of the problems associated with oestrogen deficiency. They may also help to relieve some of the more unpleasant symptoms. They include nutritional therapies, vitamins, essential fatty acids, minerals and amino acids. To protect against osteoporosis have a look for the special formulations for bones that contain calcium and vitamin D together with other minerals. A good multivitamin supplement can also help to maintain healthy levels of all body nutrients to ensure that everything works as it should. Vitamin B6 has been recommended for women that had pre-menstrual syndrome and is also useful for women going through the menopause. Remember that the two conditions are caused by the same hormone, oestrogen. Essential fatty acids can be obtained from starflower and evening primrose oil supplements.

WHAT DOES THAT WORD MEAN?

ABDOMEN - the area of the belly, between the bottom of the ribs and the groin.

BONE DENSITY - a measure of the amount of mineral, mainly calcium, in a bone.

BONE LOSS - the process of losing bone density.

CANCER - a disease that is caused by the rapid multiplication of abnormal cells in any part of the body.

CARDIOVASCULAR DISEASE - any disease of the circulatory system.

CERVICAL SMEAR - a test performed to check for abnormal changes to the cells on the cervix.

CHOLESTEROL - a steroid that is classified as a lipid that is a constituent of all animal cells. High blood cholesterol levels increases the likelihood of cardiovascular disease.

CIRCULATION - the movement of blood around the body, via veins and arteries.

CLIMACTERIC - the years of the menopause, starting with the peri-menopause. Typically when you start experiencing menopausal symptoms.

CONTINUOUS-COMBINED HRT - a form of HRT where you take both oestrogen and progesterone.

CONTRA-INDICATIONS - the reasons for not using a particular treatment, usually because it will be made worse through side effects.

COLLAGEN - a fibrous protein that gives strength and elasticity to skin, bones, cartilage and connective tissues.

CORTICAL BONE - the hard outer layer of the bone.

D&C - dilation and curettage

DILATION AND CURETTAGE - the procedure of scraping away the lining of the uterus, under general anaesthetic.

DOWAGERS HUMP - a curve on the upper spine as a result of compression of the spinal column, often a symptom of Osteoporosis.

ENDOCRINE SYSTEM - manufactures and distributes hormones into the bloodstream.

ENDOMETRIAL ABLATION - removal of the inner lining of the uterus by the use of radio waves or laser treatment.

ENDOMETRIAL CANCER - cancer of the lining of the uterus.

ENDOMETRIOSIS - occurs when cells of the endometrium appear outside the uterus, resulting in blood blisters.

ENDOMETRIUM - the lining of the uterus.

ERT- the American spelling of HRT

ESTROGEN- the American spelling of Oestrogen.

ENZYME - proteins that cause chemical changes in other cells. They are necessary to breakdown or metabolize nutrients, drugs and hormones.

FALLOPIAN TUBES - the tubes connecting the ovaries to the uterus.

FIBROIDS - non-cancerous growths in the wall of the uterus.

GYNAECOLOGIST - a doctor specialising in diagnosis and treatment of disorders of the female genital organs.

HDL's - High Density Lipoproteins.

HIGH DENSITY LIPOPROTEINS - a form of cholesterol that attaches to low density lipoproteins and allows them to be absorbed out of blood vessels.

HORMONES - substances made by the body that are transported by the blood to affect other parts of the body.

HORMONE REPLACEMENT THERAPY- the replacement of natural hormones by manufactured hormones.

HOT FLUSH - sudden flow of heat to the skin, usually the face.

HRT- Hormone Replacement Therapy

HYPOTHALMUS - the area of the brain regulating temperature, appetite, thirst and hormonal glands. Located at the base of the brain and connected to the pituitary gland.

HYSTERECTOMY- the surgical removal of the uterus/uterus

IMPLANT - a form of HRT in which a small pellet is inserted under the skin, usually in the abdomen.

INSOMNIA - inability to sleep.

LIBIDO - sex drive.

LDL's - Low Density Lipoproteins

LOW DENSITY LIPOPROTEINS - a form of cholesterol that can become attached the the walls of blood vessels , inhibiting the flow of blood.

MENOPAUSAL - refers to the menopause

MENOPAUSE - the final menstrual period.

MENSTRUATION - the monthly (usually) bleed.

MINERALS - inorganic chemicals , essential to cellular function.

NATURAL MENOPAUSE - menopause that occurs naturally.

SURGICAL MENOPAUSE - menopause that occurs following a hysterectomy and/or removal of the ovaries.

OESTRADIOL - the most potent natural oestrogen found in the blood.

OESTROGEN- the female sex hormone, secreted mainly by the ovaries, responsible for female development.

OESTROGEN DEFICIENT - does not produce enough oestrogen.

OESTROGEN RECEPTORS - the areas of the brain that respond the presence of oestrogen.

OESTRIOL - the weakest natural oestrogen found in the blood.

OESTRONE - natural oestrogen found in the blood.

OOPHORECTOMY - removal of the ovaries (unilateral - one ovary or bilateral - both ovaries).

ORAL HRT - tablets.

OSTEOBLASTS - cells within the bone that form new bone by a constant process of rebuild and repair.

OSTEOCLASTS - cells within the bone that dissolve old bone so that it can be replaced

OSTEOPOROSIS - a disease where the bone becomes so porous, brittle and fragile that it breaks easily.

OVARIES - two organs on either side of the uterus that produce the hormone oestrogen and eggs for fertilisation.

PALPITATIONS - rapid or irregular heartbeats.

PATCH - an adhesive patch applied to the buttock or top of leg, so that HRT can be absorbed by the skin.

PEAK BONE MASS - the period when the bones contain the most mineral, usually achieved around the age of 30 - 35.

PELVIC FLOOR MUSCLES - muscles at the base of the pelvis, that support the pelvic organs.

PERI-MENOPAUSE - time before the menopause when the production of female sex hormones is reduced.

PITUATARY GLAND - gland in the brain that manufactures hormones controlling other glands.

POST-MENOPAUSE - after the final period.

PREMATURE MENOPAUSE - a menopause that occurs before the age of 45 , either naturally or surgically.

PROGESTERONE - a naturally occurring female hormone.

PROLAPSE - abnormal dropping of an organ, usually the rectum, uterus, vagina or bowel.

RDA - Recommended Daily Allowance.

RECOMMENDED DAILY ALLOWANCE - daily intake of vitamins and minerals recommended by government health agencies.

ROUTE - in this case means the way that HRT is administered.

SEX HORMONE BINDING GLOBULIN - a protein in the blood that binds with, and transports, sex hormones.

STROKE - when blood supply to the brain is affected so that normal function is reduced.

SUBCUTANEOUS HRT - an implant, usually in the lower abdomen or bottom.

SURGICAL MENOPAUSE - a menopause occurring following surgery, usually hysterectomy or removal of ovaries.

TACHYPHYLAXIS - this is a condition where some women taking subcutaneous HRT have a return of menopausal symptoms even though blood oestrogen levels are normal.

TESTOSTERONE- male sex hormone, small amounts are produced in women by the ovaries.

THROMBOSIS- blood clots that form in veins or arteries.

TRABECULAR BONE - the inner layer of bone that is most at risk from osteoporosis.

TRANSDERMAL HRT - hrt which is administered via the skin, either by patch or cream.

UTERUS - uterus

VAGINA - the birth canal, leads from the uterus to outside the body.

VASOMOTOR SYMPTOMS - symptoms of menopause that are caused by constriction of the blood vessels, hot flushes, night sweats and some headaches.

SUPPORT ORGANISATIONS

British Heart Foundation (The)
14 Fitzhardinge Street, London, W1H 6DH
Health Information Line: 08450 70 80 70

Cancer BACUP
3 Bath Place, Rivington Street, London, EC2A 3JR
Cancer information service: 0171 613 2121
Web site: http://www.cancerbacup.org.uk/

Femisa – Fibroid Embolisation: Information Support and Advice
Email: help@femisa.org.uk
Web site: www.femisa.org.uk

Gynae-C
1 Bolingbroke Road, Swindon, Wiltshire, SN2 2LB
Email: gynae_c@yahoo.com
Web site: www.gynae-c.ndo.co.uk/

Health Information Service
Telephone: 0800 66 55 44
This is a national service that has local centres. Offers information on a wide range of health related issues.

Hysterectomy Association (The)
2 Princes Court, Puddletown, Dorchester, Dorset, DT2 8UE
Web Site: www.hysterectomy-association.org.uk

Medicines and Healthcare products Regulatory Agency
Market Towers, 1 Nine Elms Lane, London SW8 5NQ,
Telephone: 020-7084 2000, fax 020-7084 2353
Email: info@mhra.gsi.gov.uk

National Endometriosis Society
Suite 50, Westminster Palace Gardens, 1-7 Artillery Row, London, SW1P 1RL
Telephone: 0808 808 2227 / 020 7222 2781

NICE, National Institute of Clinical Effectiveness
MidCity Place, 71 High Holborn, London, WC1V 6NA
Telephone 020 7067 5800
Email nice@nice.nhs.uk.
Web Site: www.nice.org.uk

National Osteoporosis Society
PO Box 10, Barton Meade House, Radstock, BATH, BA3 3YB
Telephone: 01761 432472
Fax: 01761 471104 / Helpline: 01761 472721

The SHE Trust (Simply Holistic Endometriosis)
14 Moorland Way, Lincoln, LN6 7JW
Telephone: 0870 7743665 / 4
Web Site: www.shetrust.org.uk

Women's Health
52 Featherstone Street, LONDON, EC1Y 8RT.
Telephone: 020 7251 6580

OTHER RESOURCES

There are many books and other resources available to help you in your quest for information. Please visit The Hysterectomy Association's web site for more information. You can find the site at:

http://www.hysterectomy-association.org.uk

The Woman's Guide to Hysterectomy: Expectations and Options Revised.
By Adelaide Hass and Susan L Puretz
Published by Celestial Arts; ISBN: 1587611058

Hysterectomy: What It Is and How to Cope with It Successfully (Overcoming Common Problems)
By Suzie Hayman
Published by Sheldon Press; ISBN: 085969870X

No More Hysterectomies
By Vicki Hufnagel
Published by G P Putnam's Sons; ISBN: 0452262550

Understanding Hysterectomy
By N Langford-Wood
Published by John Wiley and Sons Ltd; ISBN: 0470865318

Is It Me or Is It Hot in Here?: A Modern Woman's Guide to the Menopause
By Jenni Murray
Published by Vermilion; ISBN: 0091887771

Eat Your Way Through the Menopause
By Marilyn Glenville
Published by Kyle Cathie; ISBN: 1856264688

Menopause and the Mind: The Complete Guide to Coping with the Cognitive Effects of Perimenopause and Menopause
By Claire Warga
Published by Touchstone Books; ISBN: 0684854791.

Smart Medicine for Menopause: Hormone Replacement Therapy and Its Natural Alternatives
By Sandra Cabot
Published by Putnam Pub Group (P); ISBN: 089529897X

Alternatives to Hormone Replacement Therapy
Natural Choices for Menopause: Safe, Effective Alternatives to Hormone Replacement Therapy
By Marilyn Glenville
Published by St. Martin's Press; ISBN: 031297013.

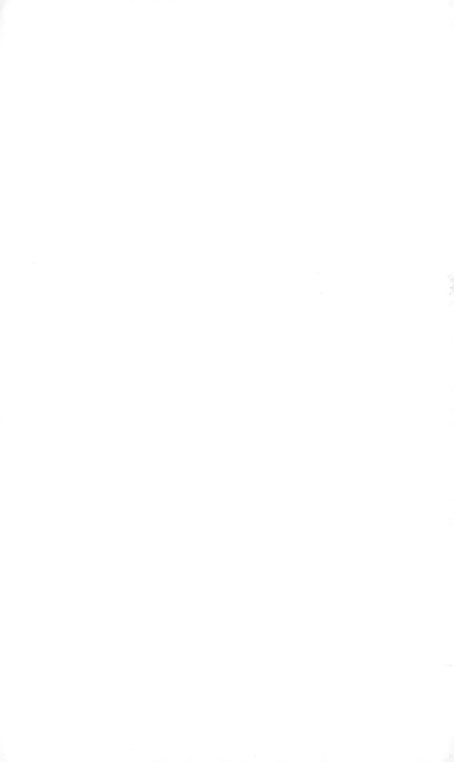

33409479R00046

Printed in Great Britain
by Amazon